My air Fryer Everyday Dessert

Tasty and Incredibly Healthy Desserts to Enjoy Your Diet and Lose Weight

Franck McMillan

TABLE OF CONTENT

this book has been derived from various sources. Please consult a licensed professional before attempting any techniques outlined in this book.

By reading this document, the reader agrees that under no circumstances is the author responsible for any losses, direct or indirect, which are incurred as a result of the use of information contained within this document, including, but not limited to, — errors, omissions, or inaccuracies.

Easy Baked Chocolate Mug Cake

Preparation Time:5 minutes

Cooking Time: 15 minutes

Servings: 3

Ingredients:

- ½ cup cocoa powder
- ½ cup stevia powder
- 1 cup coconut cream
- 1 package cream cheese, room temperature
- 1 tablespoon vanilla extract
- tablespoons butter

Directions:

1. Preheat the air fryer oven for 5 minutes.
2. In a mixing bowl, combine all ingredients.
3. Use a hand mixer to mix everything until fluffy.
4. Pour into greased mugs.
5. Place the mugs in the fryer basket.
6. Bake for 15 minutes at 350°f.
7. Place in the fridge to chill before serving.

Nutrition: Calories: 744 Fat:69.7g protein:13.9g

sugar:4g

Fried Peaches

Preparation Time:2 hours 10 minutes

Cooking Time: 15 minutes

Servings: 4

Ingredients:

- 4 ripe peaches (1/2 a peach = 1 serving)
- 1/2 cups flour
- Salt
- egg yolks
- 3/4 cups cold water
- 1/2 tablespoons olive oil
- tablespoons brandy
- egg whites
- Cinnamon/sugar mix

Directions:

1. Mix flour, egg yolks, and salt in a mixing bowl. Slowly mix in water, then add brandy. Set the mixture aside for 2 hours and go do something for 1 hour 45 minutes.

2. Boil a large pot of water and cut and x at the bottom of each peach. While the water boils fill another large bowl with water and

ice. Boil each peach for about a minute, then plunge it in the ice bath. Now the peels should basically fall off the peach. Beat the egg whites and mix into the batter mix. Dip each peach in the mix to coat.

3. Pour the coated peach into the oven rack/basket. Place the rack on the middle-shelf of the air fryer oven. Set temperature to 360°f, and set Time to 10 minutes.

4. Directions: are a plate with cinnamon/sugar mix, roll peaches in mix and serve.

Nutrition: Calories: 306 Fat:3g protein:10g fiber:2.7g

Apple Dumplings

Preparation Time:10 minutes

Cooking Time: 25 minutes

Servings: 4

Ingredients:

- 2 tbsp. Melted coconut oil
- 2 puff pastry sheets
- tbsp. Brown sugar
- tbsp. Raisins
- small apples of choice

Directions:

1. Ensure your air fryer oven is preheated to 356 degrees.
2. Core and peel apples and mix with raisins and sugar.
3. Place a bit of apple mixture into puff pastry sheets and brush sides with melted coconut oil.
4. Place into the air fryer. Cook 25 minutes, turning halfway through. Will be golden when done.

Nutrition: Calories: 367 Fat:7g protein:2g sugar:5g

Air Fryer Chocolate Cake

Preparation Time: 5 minutes

Cooking Time: 35 minutes

Servings: 8-10

Ingredients:

- ½ c. Hot water
- tsp. Vanilla
- ¼ c. Olive oil
- ½ c. Almond milk
- egg
- ½ tsp. Salt
- ¾ tsp. Baking soda
- ¾ tsp. Baking powder
- ½ c. Unsweetened cocoa powder
- c. Almond flour
- 1 c. Brown sugar

Directions:

- Preheat your air fryer oven to 356 degrees.
- Stir all dry ingredients together. Then stir in wet ingredients. Add hot water last.
- The batter will be thin, no worries.

- Pour cake batter into a pan that fits into the fryer. Cover with foil and poke holes into the foil.
- Bake 35 minutes.
- Discard foil and then bake another 10 minutes.

Nutrition: Calories: 378 Fat:9g protein:4g sugar:5g

Banana-Choco Brownies

Preparation Time:5 minutes

Cooking Time: 30 minutes

Servings: 12

Ingredients:

- 2 cups almond flour
- 2 teaspoons baking powder
- ½ teaspoon baking powder
- ½ teaspoon baking soda
- ½ teaspoon salt
- over-ripe banana
- large eggs
- ½ teaspoon stevia powder
- ¼ cup coconut oil
- 1 tablespoon vinegar
- 1/3 cup almond flour
- 1/3 cup cocoa powder

Directions:

1. Preheat the air fryer oven for 5 minutes.
2. Combine all ingredients in a food processor and pulse until well-combined.
3. Pour into a baking dish that will fit in the air fryer.

4. Place in the air fryer basket and cook for 30 minutes at 350°f or if a toothpick inserted in the middle comes out clean.

Nutrition: Calories: 75 Fat:6.5g protein:1.7g sugar:2g

Easy Air Fryer Donuts

Preparation Time:5 minutes

Cooking Time: 5 minutes

Servings: 8

Ingredients:

- Pinch of allspice
- 4 tbsp. Dark brown sugar
- ½ - 1 tsp. Cinnamon
- 1/3 c. Granulated sweetener
- 3 tbsp. Melted coconut oil
- can of biscuits

Directions:

1. Mix allspice, sugar, sweetener, and cinnamon together.
2. Take out biscuits from can and with a circle cookie cutter, cut holes from centers and place into air fryer.
3. Cook 5 minutes at 350 degrees. As batches are cooked, use a brush to coat with melted coconut oil and dip each into sugar mixture.
4. Serve warm!

Nutrition: Calories: 209 Fat:4g protein:0g sugar:3g

Chocolate Souffle For Two

Preparation Time:5 minutes

Cooking Time: 14 minutes

Servings: 2

Ingredients:

- 2 tbsp. Almond flour
- ½ tsp. Vanilla
- 3 tbsp. Sweetener
- 2 separated eggs
- ¼ c. Melted coconut oil
- 3 ounces of semi-sweet chocolate, chopped

Directions:

1. Brush coconut oil and sweetener onto ramekins.
2. Melt coconut oil and chocolate together.
3. Beat egg yolks well, adding vanilla and sweetener. Stir in flour and ensure there are no lumps.
4. Preheat the air fryer oven to 330 degrees.
5. Whisk egg whites till they reach peak state and fold them into chocolate mixture.

6. Pour batter into ramekins and place into the air fryer oven.
7. Cook 14 minutes.
8. Serve with powdered sugar dusted on top.

Nutrition: Calories: 238 Fat:6g protein:1g sugar:4g

Fried Bananas with Chocolate Sauce

Preparation Time:10 minutes

Cooking Time: 10 minutes

Servings: 2

Ingredients:

- large egg
- ¼ cup cornstarch
- ¼ cup plain bread crumbs
- bananas, halved crosswise
- Cooking oil
- Chocolate sauce (see ingredient tip)

Directions:

1. In a small bowl, beat the egg. In another bowl, place the cornstarch. Place the bread crumbs in a third bowl. Dip the bananas in the cornstarch, then the egg
2. and then the bread crumbs.
3. Spray the air fryer basket with cooking oil. Place the bananas in the basket and spray them with cooking oil.
4. Set temperature to 360°f and cook for 5 minutes. Open the air fryer and flip the

bananas. Cook for an additional 2 minutes. Transfer the bananas to plates.

5. Drizzle the chocolate sauce over the bananas, and serve.

6. You can make your own chocolate sauce using 2 tablespoons milk and ¼ cup chocolate chips. Heat a saucepan over medium-high heat. Add the milk and stir for 1 to 2 minutes. Add the chocolate chips. Stir for 2 minutes, or until the chocolate has melted.

Nutrition: Calories: 203 Fat:6g protein:3g fiber:3g

Apple Hand Pies

Preparation Time:5 minutes

Cooking Time: 8 minutes

Servings: 6

Ingredients:

- 15-ounces no-sugar-added apple pie filling
- store-bought crust

Directions:

1. Lay out pie crust and slice into equal-sized squares.
2. Place 2 tbsp. Filling into each square and seal crust with a fork.
3. Pour into the oven rack/basket. Place the rack on the middle-shelf of the air fryer oven. Set temperature to 390°f, and set Time to 8 minutes until golden in color.

Nutrition: Calories: 278 Fat:10g protein:5g sugar:4g

Chocolaty Banana Muffins

Preparation Time:5 minutes

Cooking Time: 25 minutes

Servings: 12

Ingredients:

- ¾ cup whole wheat flour
- ¾ cup plain flour
- ¼ cup cocoa powder
- ¼ teaspoon baking powder
- teaspoon baking soda
- ¼ teaspoon salt
- large bananas, peeled and mashed
- 1 cup sugar
- 1/3 cup canola oil
- 1 egg
- ½ teaspoon vanilla essence
- 1 cup mini chocolate chips

Directions:

1. In a large bowl, mix together flour, cocoa powder, baking powder, baking soda and salt.

2. In another bowl, add bananas, sugar, oil, egg and vanilla extract and beat till well combined.

3. Slowly, add flour mixture in egg mixture and mix till just combined.

4. Fold in chocolate chips.

5. Preheat the air fryer oven to 345 degrees f. Grease 12 muffin molds.

6. Transfer the mixture into muffin molds evenly and cook for about 20-25 minutes or till a toothpick inserted in the center comes out clean.

7. Remove the muffin molds from air fryer and keep on wire rack to cool for about 10 minutes. Carefully turn on a wire rack to cool completely before serving.

Nutrition: Calories: 203 Fat:6g protein:3g fiber:3g

Blueberry Lemon Muffins

Preparation Time:5 minutes

Cooking Time: 10 minutes

Servings: 12

Ingredients:

- tsp. Vanilla
- Juice and zest of 1 lemon
- eggs
- c. Blueberries
- ½ c. Cream
- ¼ c. Avocado oil
- ½ c. Monk fruit
- ½ c. Almond flour

Directions:

- mix monk fruit and flour together.
- In another bowl, mix vanilla, egg
- lemon juice, and cream together. Add mixtures together and blend well.
- Spoon batter into cupcake holders.
- place in air fryer oven. Bake 10 minutes at 320 degrees, checking at 6 minutes to ensure you don't overbake them.

Nutrition: Calories: 317   Fat:11g   protein:3g

sugar:5g

Sweet Cream Cheese Wontons

Preparation Time:5 minutes

Cooking Time: 5 minutes

Servings: 16

Ingredients:

- egg mixed with a bit of water
- Wonton wrappers
- ½ c. Powdered erythritol
- 8 ounces softened cream cheese
- Olive oil

Directions:

1. Mix sweetener and cream cheese together.
2. Lay out 4 wontons at a Time and cover with a dish towel to prevent drying out.
3. Place ½ of a teaspoon of cream cheese mixture into each wrapper.
4. Dip finger into egg/water mixture and fold diagonally to form a triangle. Seal edges well.
5. Repeat with remaining ingredients.

6. Place filled wontons into the air fryer oven
   and cook 5 minutes at 400 degrees,
   shaking halfway through cooking.

Nutrition: Calories: 303 Fat:3g protein:0.5g sugar:4g

Air Fryer Cinnamon Rolls

Preparation Time:15 minutes

Cooking Time: 5 minutes

Servings: 8

Ingredients:

- ¾ c. Brown sugar
- ¼ c. Melted coconut oil
- 1-pound frozen bread dough, thawed
- Glaze:
- ½ tsp. Vanilla
- 1 ¼ c. Powdered erythritol
- tbsp. Softened ghee
- Ounces softened cream cheese

Directions:

1. Lay out bread dough and roll out into a rectangle. Brush melted ghee over dough and leave a 1-inch border along edges.
2. Mix cinnamon and sweetener together and then sprinkle over dough.
3. Roll dough tightly and slice into 8 pieces. Let sit 1-2 hours to rise.
4. To make the glaze, simply mix ingredients together till smooth.

5. Once rolls rise, place into air fryer and cook 5 minutes at 350 degrees.

6. Serve rolls drizzled in cream cheese glaze. Enjoy!

Nutrition: Calories: 390 Fat:8g protein:1g sugar:7g

Bread Pudding with Cranberry

Preparation Time:5 minutes

Cooking Time: 45 minutes

Servings: 4

Ingredients:

- 1-1/2 cups milk
- 2-1/2 eggs
- 1/2 cup cranberries1 teaspoon butter
- 1/4 cup and 2 tablespoons white sugar
- 1/4 cup golden raisins
- 1/8 teaspoon ground cinnamon
- 3/4 cup heavy whipping cream
- 3/4 teaspoon lemon zest
- 3/4 teaspoon kosher salt
- 3/4 French baguettes, cut into 2-inch slices
- 3/8 vanilla bean, split and seeds scraped away

Directions:

1. Lightly grease baking pan of air fryer with cooking spray. Spread baguette slices, cranberries, and raisins.

2. In blender, blend well vanilla bean, cinnamon, salt, lemon zest, eggs, sugar, and cream. Pour over baguette slices. Let it soak for an hour.

3. Cover pan with foil.

4. For 35 minutes, cook on 330°f.

5. Let it rest for 10 minutes.

6. Serve and enjoy.

Nutrition: Calories: 581 Fat:23.8g protein:15.8g sugar:7g

Easy Cheesecake

Preparation Time:10 minutes

Cooking Time: 10 minutes

Servings:6

Ingredients:

- 2 eggs
- 16 oz cream cheese, softened
- 2 tbsp sour cream
- 1/2 tsp fresh lemon juice
- tsp vanilla
- 3/4 cup erythritol

Instructions:

1. Preheat the air fryer to 350 f.
2. Add eggs, lemon juice, vanilla, and sweetener in a large bowl and beat using a hand mixer until smooth.
3. Add cream cheese and sour cream and beat until fluffy.
4. Pour batter into the 2 four-inch spring-form pan and place in air fryer basket and cook for 8-10minutes at 350 f.
5. Remove from air fryer and let it cool completely.

6. Place in refrigerator for overnight.

7. Serve and enjoy.

Nutrition: Calories: 367 Protein: 2 g. Fat: 7 g. Carbs: 10 g.

Fluffy Butter Cake

Preparation Time:10 minutes

Cooking Time: 35 minutes

Servings:8

Ingredients:

- 6egg yolks
- 3cups almond flour
- 2tsp vanilla
- 1egg, lightly beaten
- ¼ cup erythritol
- 1cup butter
- Pinch of salt

Directions:

1. Preheat the air fryer to 350 F.
2. In a bowl, beat butter and sweetener until fluffy.
3. Add vanilla, egg yolks and beat until well combined.
4. Add remaining ingredients and beat until combined.
5. Pour batter into air fryer cake pan and place into the air fryer and cook for 35 minutes.
6. Slice and serve.

Nutrition: Calories: 212 Protein: 7 g. Fat: 8 g. Carbs: 13 g.

Ricotta Lemon Cake

Preparation Time:10 minutes

Cooking Time: 40 minutes

Servings:8

Ingredients:

- 1lb ricotta
- 4eggs
- 1lemon juice
- 1lemon zest
- ¼ cup erythritol

Directions:

1. Preheat the air fryer to 325 F.
2. Spray air fryer baking dish with cooking spray.
3. In a bowl, beat ricotta cheese until smooth.
4. Whisk in the eggs one by one.
5. Whisk in lemon juice and zest.
6. Pour batter into the baking dish and place into the air fryer.
7. Cook for 40 minutes.
8. Allow to cool completely then slice and serve.

Nutrition: Calories: 367 Protein: 2 g. Fat: 7 g. Carbs:

10 g.

Sponge Cake

Preparation Time:10 minutes

Cooking Time: 40 minutes

Servings:12

Ingredients:

- 4eggs
- ½ cup swerve
- 2cups almond flour
- 1tsp vanilla
- 1cup margarine

Directions:

1. Preheat the air fryer to 350 F.
2. Spray air fryer cake pan with cooking spray and set aside.
3. In a large bowl, beat margarine and sweetener using a hand mixer until light and fluffy.
4. Add egg one by one and beat well.
5. Add vanilla and almond flour and mix until well combined.
6. Pour batter into the pan and place into the air fryer.
7. Cook for 40 minutes.

8. Slice and serve.

Nutrition: Calories: 140 Protein: 2 g. Fat: 0 g. Carbs: 5 g.

Almond Coconut Lemon Cake

Preparation Time:10 minutes

Cooking Time: 48 minutes

Servings:10

Ingredients:

- 4 eggs
- 2tbsp lemon zest
- 1/2cup butter softened
- 2tsp baking powder
- 1/4cup coconut flour
- 2cups almond flour
- 1/2 cup fresh lemon juice
- 1/4cup swerve
- 1tbsp vanilla

Directions:

1. Preheat the air fryer to 280 F.
2. Spray air fryer baking dish with cooking spray and set aside.
3. In a large bowl, beat all Ingredients: using a hand mixer until a smooth.
4. Pour batter into the dish and place into the air fryer and cook for 48 minutes.

5. Slice and serve.

Nutrition: Calories: 212 Protein: 7 g. Fat: 8 g. Carbs: 13 g.

Vanilla Butter Cheese Cake

Preparation Time:10 minutes

Cooking Time: 32 minutes

Servings:9

Ingredients:

- 5 eggs
- 1cup erythritol
- 4oz cream cheese, softened
- 1tsp vanilla
- 1tsp baking powder
- 6.5oz almond flour
- 1/2 cup butter, softened

Directions:

1. Preheat the air fryer to 325 F.
2. Spray air fryer cake pan with cooking spray and set aside.
3. Add all Ingredients into the large bowl and beat until fluffy.
4. Pour batter into the pan and place into the air fryer and cook for 32 minutes.
5. Slice and serve.

Nutrition: Calories: 367 Protein: 2 g. Fat: 7 g. Carbs: 10 g.

Almond Cinnamon Mug Cake

Preparation Time:5 minutes

Cooking Time: 10 minutes

Servings:1

Ingredients:

- 1scoop vanilla protein powder
- 1/2 tsp cinnamon
- 1tsp granulated sweetener
- 1tbsp almond flour
- 1/2 tsp baking powder
- 1/4 tsp vanilla
- 1/4 cup unsweetened almond milk

Directions:

1. Add protein powder, cinnamon, almond flour, sweetener, and baking powder into the mug and mix well.
2. Add vanilla and almond milk and stir well.
3. Place mug in the air fryer and cook at 390 F for 10 minutes
4. Serve and enjoy.

Nutrition: Calories: 140 Protein: 2 g. Fat: 0 g. Carbs: 5 g.

Chocolate Coconut Cake

Preparation Time:10 minutes

Cooking Time: 20 minutes

Servings:9

Ingredients:

- 6 eggs
- 2 tsp baking powder
- 3 oz unsweetened cocoa powder
- 5 oz erythritol
- oz coconut flour
- tsp vanilla
- oz butter, melted
- 11 oz heavy cream

Directions:

1. Preheat the air fryer to 325 F.
2. In a bowl, mix together coconut flour, butter, 5 oz heavy cream, eggs, baking powder half cocoa powder, and 3 oz sweetener until well combined.
3. Pour batter into the greased cake pan and place into the air fryer and cook for 20 minutes.
4. Allow to cool completely.

5. In a large bowl, beat remaining heavy cream, cocoa powder, and sweetener until smooth.

6. Spread the cream on top of cake and place in the refrigerator for 30 minutes.

7. Slice and serve.

Nutrition: Calories: 212 Protein: 7 g. Fat: 8 g. Carbs: 13 g.

Choco Fudge Cake

Preparation Time:10 minutes

Cooking Time: 24 minutes

Servings:12

Ingredients:

- 6 eggs
- 1/2 cup swerve
- oz unsweetened chocolate, melted
- 1/2 cup almond flour
- oz butter, melted Pinch of salt

Directions:

1. Preheat the air fryer to 325 F.
2. Spray air fryer cake pan with cooking spray and set aside.
3. In a large bowl, beat eggs until foamy. Add sweetener and stir well.
4. Add melted butter, chocolate, almond flour, and salt and stir to combine.
5. Pour batter into the pan and place into the air fryer and cook for 24 minutes.
6. Slice and serve.

Nutrition: Calories: 367 Protein: 2 g. Fat: 7 g. Carbs: 10 g.

Cranberry Almond Cake

Preparation Time:10 minutes

Cooking Time: 16 minutes

Servings:6

Ingredients:

- 4 eggs
- 1tsp orange zest
- 2tsp mixed spice
- 2 tsp cinnamon
- 1/4 cup swerve
- cup butter, softened
- 2/3 cup dried cranberries
- 1/2 cups almond flour
- 1 tsp vanilla

Directions:

1. Preheat the air fryer to 325 F.
2. In a bowl, add sweetener and melted butter and beat until fluffy.
3. Add cinnamon, vanilla, and mixed spice and stir well.
4. Add eggs stir until well combined.
5. Add almond flour, orange zest, and cranberries and stir to combine.

6. Pour batter in a greased air fryer cake pan and place into the air fryer.

7. Cook cake for 16 minutes.

8. Slice and serve.

Nutrition: Calories: 140 Protein: 2 g. Fat: 0 g. Carbs: 5 g.

Pumpkin Custard

Preparation Time:10 minutes

Cooking Time: 32 minutes

Servings:6

Ingredients:

- 4 egg yolks
- 1/2 tsp cinnamon
- 15 drops liquid stevia
- 15 oz pumpkin puree
- 3/4 cup coconut cream
- 1/8 tsp cloves
- 1/8 tsp ginger

Directions:

1. Preheat the air fryer to 325 F.
2. In a large bowl, combine together pumpkin puree, cinnamon, swerve, cloves, and ginger.
3. Add egg yolks and beat until combined.
4. Add coconut cream and stir well.
5. Pour mixture into the six ramekins and place into the air fryer.
6. Cook for 32 minutes.

7. Let it cool completely then place in the refrigerator.

8. Serve chilled and enjoy.

Nutrition: Calories: 170 Protein: 4 g. Fat: 1 g. Carbs: 6 g.

Angel Food Cake

Preparation Time:5 minutes

Cooking Time: 30 minutes

Servings: 12

Ingredients:

- ¼ cup butter, melted
- cup powdered erythritol
- teaspoon strawberry extract
- 12 egg whites
- teaspoons cream of tartar

Directions:

1. Preheat the air fryer oven for 5 minutes. Blend the cream of tartar and egg whites.
2. Use a hand mixer and whisk until white and fluffy.
3. Add the rest of the ingredients except for the butter and whisk for another minute.
4. Pour into a baking dish.
5. Place in the air fryer basket and cook for 30 minutes at 400°F or if a toothpick inserted in the middle comes out clean.
6. Drizzle with melted butter once cooled.

Nutrition: Calories: 65 Protein: 3.1 g. Fat: 5 g. Carbs:

6.2 g.

Strawberry Cheese Cake

Preparation Time:10 minutes

Cooking Time: 35 minutes

Servings:6

Ingredients:

- 1cup almond flour
- 3tbsp coconut oil, melted
- ½ tsp vanilla
- 1egg, lightly beaten
- 1tbsp fresh lime juice
- ¼ cup erythritol
- 1cup cream cheese, softened
- 1lb strawberries, chopped
- 2tsp baking powder

Directions:

1. Add all Ingredients into the large bowl and mix until well combined.
2. Spray air fryer cake pan with cooking spray.
3. Pour batter into the pan and place into the air fryer and cook at 350 F for 35 minutes.
4. Allow to cool completely.

Nutrition: Calories: 140 Protein: 2 g. Fat: 0 g. Carbs:

5 g.

Easy Orange Coconut Cake

Preparation Time:5 minutes

Cooking Time: 17 minutes

Serves 6

Ingredients:

- stick butter, melted
- ¾ cup granulated Swerve
- eggs, beaten
- ¾ cup coconut flour
- ¼ teaspoon salt
- 1/3 teaspoon grated nutmeg
- 1/3 cup coconut milk
- 1/4cups almond flour
- ½ teaspoon baking powder
- tablespoons unsweetened orange jam
- Cooking spray

Directions:

1. Coat a baking pan with cooking spray. Set aside.
2. In a large mixing bowl, whisk together the melted butter and granulated Swerve until fluffy.

3. Mix in the beaten eggs and whisk again until smooth. Stir in the salt, nutmeg, and coconut flour and gradually pour in the coconut milk. Add the remaining ingredients and stir until well incorporated.

4. Scrape the batter into the baking pan.

5. Place the pan on the bake position.

6. Select Bake, set temperature to 355ºF (179ºC), and set Time to 17 minutes.

7. When cooking is complete, the top of the cake should spring back when gently pressed with your fingers.

8. Remove from the air fryer grill to a wire rack to cool. Serve chilled.

Nutrition: Calories: 367 Protein: 2 g. Fat: 7 g. Carbs: 10 g.

Easy Lava Cake

Preparation Time:10 minutes

Cooking Time: 9 minutes

Servings:2

Ingredients:

- egg
- ½ tsp baking powder
- tbsp coconut oil, melted
- tbsp flax meal2 tbsp erythritol
- Tbsp water
- tbsp unsweetened cocoa powder pinch of salt

Directions:

1. Whisk all Ingredients into the bowl and transfer in two ramekins.
2. Preheat the air fryer to 350 f.
3. Place ramekins in air fryer basket and bake for 8-9 minutes.
4. Carefully remove ramekins from air fryer and let it cool for 10 minutes.
5. Serve and enjoy.

Nutrition: Calories: 65 Protein: 3.1 g. Fat: 5 g. Carbs: 6.2 g.

Choco Mug Cake

Preparation Time:5 minutes

Cooking Time: 20 minutes

Servings:1

Ingredients:

- 1egg, lightly beaten
- 1tbsp heavy cream
- ¼ tsp baking powder
- 2tbsp unsweetened cocoa powder
- 2tbsp erythritol
- ½tsp vanilla
- 1tbsp peanut butter
- 1tsp salt

Directions:

1. Preheat the air fryer to 400 f.
2. In a bowl, mix together all ingredients until well combined.
3. Spray mug with cooking spray.
4. Pour batter in mug and place in the air fryer and cook for 20 minutes.
5. Serve and enjoy.

Nutrition: Calories: 212 Protein: 7 g. Fat: 8 g. Carbs: 13 g.

Egg Custard

Preparation Time:10 minutes

Cooking Time: 32 minutes

Servings:6

Ingredients:

- 2 egg yolks
- 3 eggs
- 1/2 cup erythritol
- 2 cups heavy whipping cream
- 1/2 tsp vanilla
- tsp nutmeg

Directions:

1. Preheat the air fryer to 325 F.
2. Add all Ingredients into the large bowl and beat until well combined.
3. Pour custard mixture into the greased baking dish and place into the air fryer.
4. Cook for 32 minutes.
5. Let it cool completely then place in the refrigerator for 1-2 hours.
6. Serve and enjoy.

Nutrition: Calories: 170 Protein: 4 g. Fat: 1 g. Carbs: 6 g

Chocolate Custard

Preparation Time:10 minutes

Cooking Time: 32 minutes

Servings:4

Ingredients:

- 2 eggs
- tsp vanilla
- cup heavy whipping cream
- 1 cup unsweetened almond milk
- tbsp unsweetened cocoa powder
- 1/4 cup Swerve Pinch of salt

Directions:

1. Preheat the air fryer to 305 F.
2. Add all Ingredients into the blender and blend until well combined.
3. Pour mixture into the ramekins and place into the air fryer.
4. Cook for 32 minutes.
5. Serve and enjoy.

Nutrition: Calories: 212 Protein: 7 g. Fat: 8 g. Carbs: 13 g.

Delicious Vanilla Custard

Preparation Time:10 minutes

Cooking Time: 20 minutes

Servings:2

Ingredients:

- eggs
- 2 tbsp swerve
- 1tsp vanilla
- ½ cup unsweetened almond milk
- ½ cup cream cheese

Directions:

1. Add eggs in a bowl and beat using a hand mixer.
2. Add cream cheese, sweetener, vanilla, and almond milk and beat for 2 minutes more.
3. Spray two ramekins with cooking spray.
4. Pour batter into the ramekins.
5. Preheat the air fryer to 350 F.
6. Place ramekins into the air fryer and cook for 20 minutes.
7. Serve and enjoy.

Nutrition: Calories: 212 Protein: 7 g. Fat: 8 g. Carbs: 13 g.

Honey Graham Crackers Pie

Preparation Time:10 Minutes

Cooking Time: 45 Minutes

Servings: 8

Ingredients:

- 2 Cups self-rising flour
- Cup almond flour
- 1 Teaspoon baking powder
- ½ Cup butter, softened
- ½ Cup packed brown sugar
- 1/3 Cup honey
- 1 Teaspoon vanilla extract
- ½ Cup coconut milk

Directions:

1. Sieve self-rising flour, almond flour, baking powder and baking powder; keep separately. In a medium container, butter, brown sugar and honey stir gently and loosely. Add the sifted Ingredients: alternately with milk and vanilla.

2. Cover the dough and cool it overnight.
   Preheat the Air fryer toaster oven to 175°C.
   Divide the cold dough into quarters.

3. Spread the dough on a well-floured surface
   quarterly in a 5 x 15-inch rectangle. Divide
   into rectangles with a knife. Place
   rectangles on non-greased baking sheets.
   Draw a line in the middle and click with a
   fork.

4. For a cinnamon biscuit, sprinkle with a
   mixture of sugar and cinnamon before
   baking. Bake in the preheated oven for 13
   to 15 minutes. Remove the baking trays to
   cool them on racks.

Nutrition: Calories: 120 Cal Fat: 3.9 g Carbs: 1.9 g
Protein: 1.9g

Peach Pie Mix

Preparation Time: 15 minutes

Cooking Time:35 minute |

Servings: 5

Ingredients:

- tbsp of dark rum
- pie dough
- tbsp of cornstarch
- Ground nutmeg
- tbsp of butter
- 2 tbsp of flour
- 2-1/4 pound of peaches
- 1 tbsp of lemon juice
- 1/2 cup of sugar

Directions:

1. Press the dough on the Power XL Air Fryer Grill pan
2. Mix sugar, nutmeg, lemon juice, cornstarch, and butter in a bowl.
3. Add peaches, rum, and flour.
4. Mix well
5. Pour the mixture into the dough.

6. Set the Power XL Air Fryer Grill to toast/bagel function.

7. Cook for 35 minutes at 3500F.

8. Serve immediately or allow cooling before serving

9. Serving Suggestions: serve with orange juice

10. Directions: & Cooking Tips: mix Ingredients: well

Nutrition: Calories: 261kcal, Fat: 12g, Carb: 39g, Proteins: 3g

Southern Fudge Pie

Preparation Time:15 minutes

Cooking Time: 26 minutes

Serves 8

Ingredients:

- 1/2cups sugar
- 1/2cup self-rising flour
- 1/3 cup unsweetened cocoa powder
- large eggs, beaten
- 12 tablespoons (1 1/2 sticks) butter, melted
- 1 1/2teaspoons vanilla extract
- 1 (9-inch) unbaked pie crust
- 1/4cup confectioners' sugar (optional)

Directions:

1. Thoroughly combine the flour, cocoa powder, and sugar in a medium bowl. Add the beaten eggs and butter and whisk to combine. Stir in the vanilla.
2. Pour the filling into the pie crust and transfer to the air fry basket.
3. Place the basket on the bake position.

4. Select bake, set temperature to 350ºf (180ºc), and set Time to 26 minutes.

5. When cooking is complete, the pie should be set.

6. Allow the pie to cool for 5 minutes. Sprinkle with the confectioners' sugar, if desired. Serve warm.

Nutrition: Calories: 212 Protein: 7 g. Fat: 8 g. Carbs: 13 g.

Cashew Pie

Preparation Time:10 minutes

Cooking Time: 18 minutes

Servings:8

Ingredients:

- 1egg
- 2oz cashews, crushed
- ½ tsp baking soda
- 1/3 cup heavy cream
- 1oz dark chocolate, melted
- 1tbsp butter
- 1tsp vinegar
- 1cup coconut flour

Directions:

1. Add egg in a bowl and beat using a hand mixer. Add coconut flour and stir well.
2. Add butter, vinegar, baking soda, heavy cream, and melted chocolate and stir well.
3. Add cashews and mix well.
4. Preheat the air fryer to 350 f.
5. Add dough in air fryer baking dish and flatten it into a pie shape.
6. Cook for 18 minutes.

7. Slice and serve.

Nutrition: Calories: 212 Protein: 7 g. Fat: 8 g. Carbs: 13 g.

Vanilla Butter Pie

Preparation Time:10 minutes

Cooking Time: 20 minutes

Servings:8

Ingredients:

- 1egg
- 2tbsp erythritol
- ½ cup butter, melted
- 1tsp vanilla
- 1cup almond flour
- 1tsp baking soda
- 1tbsp vinegar

Directions:

1. Mix together almond flour and baking soda in a bowl.
2. In a separate bowl, whisk the egg with sweetener and vanilla.
3. Pour whisk egg, vinegar, and butter in almond flour and mix until dough is formed.
4. Preheat the air fryer to 340 f.
5. Roll dough using the rolling pin in air fryer baking dish size.

6. Place rolled dough in air fryer baking dish. Place in the air fryer and cook for 20 minutes.

7. Slice and serve.

Nutrition: Calories: 140 Protein: 2 g. Fat: 0 g. Carbs: 5 g.

Bourbon Chocolate Pecan Pie

Preparation Time:20 minutes

Cooking Time: 25 minutes

Serves 8

Ingredients:

- (9-inch) unbaked pie crust
- Filling:
- large eggs
- 1/3cup butter, melted
- cup sugar
- 1/2 cup all-purpose flour
- cup milk chocolate chips
- 1 1/2cups coarsely chopped pecans
- tablespoons bourbon

Directions:

1. Whisk the eggs and melted butter in a large bowl until creamy.
2. Add the flour and sugar and stir to incorporate. Mix in the pecans, milk chocolate chips, and bourbon and stir until well combined.

3. Use a fork to prick holes in the bottom and sides of the pie crust. Pour the filling into the pie crust. Place the pie crust in the air fry basket.

4. Place the basket on the bake position.

5. Select bake, set temperature to 350ºf (180ºc), and set Time to 25 minutes.

6. When cooking is complete, a toothpick inserted in the center should come out clean.

7. Allow the pie cool for 10 minutes in the basket before serving.

Nutrition: Calories: 140 Protein: 2 g. Fat: 0 g. Carbs: 5 g.

Chocolate Pudding

Preparation Time:10 Minutes

Cooking Time: 10 Minutes

Serves 8

Ingredients:

- egg
- egg yolk
- ¾ cup chocolate milk
- tablespoons brown sugar
- tablespoons peanut butter
- tablespoons cocoa powder
- 1 teaspoon vanilla
- slices firm white bread, cubed
- Nonstick cooking spray

Directions:

1. Spritz a baking pan with nonstick cooking spray.

2. Whisk together the egg yolk, egg, peanut butter, chocolate milk, cocoa powder, brown sugar, and vanilla until well combined.

3. Fold in the bread cubes and stir to mix well. Allow the bread soak for 10 minutes.

4. When ready, transfer the egg mixture to the baking pan.

5. Place the pan on the bake position.

6. Select bake, set temperature to 330ºf (166ºc), and set Time to 10 minutes.

7. When done, the pudding should be just firm to the touch.

8. Serve at room temperature.

Nutrition: Calories: 367 Protein: 2 g. Fat: 7 g. Carbs: 10 g.

Coconut Pie

Preparation Time:10 minutes

Cooking Time: 12 minutes

Servings:6

Ingredients:

- 2 eggs
- 1/2 cup coconut flour
- 1/2 cup erythritol
- 1cup shredded coconut
- 11/2tsp vanilla
- 1/4cup butter
- 11/2 cups coconut milk

Directions:

1. Add all Ingredients into the large bowl and mix until well combined.
2. Spray a 6-inch baking dish with cooking spray.
3. Pour batter into the dish and place in the air fryer basket.
4. Cook at 350 f for 10-12 minutes.
5. Slice and serve.

Nutrition: Calories: 212 Protein: 7 g. Fat: 8 g. Carbs: 13 g.

Pumpkin Muffins

Preparation Time:10 minutes

Cooking Time: 20 minutes

Servings:10

Ingredients:

- Large eggs
- 1/2 cup pumpkin puree
- 1tbsp pumpkin pie spice
- 1tbsp baking powder, gluten-free
- 2/3 cup erythritol
- 1tsp vanilla
- 1/3 cup coconut oil, melted
- 1/2 cup almond flour
- 1/2 cup coconut flour
- 1/2 tsp sea salt

Directions:

1. Preheat the air fryer to 325 f.
2. In a large bowl, stir together coconut flour, pumpkin pie spice, baking powder, erythritol, almond flour, and sea salt.
3. Stir in eggs, vanilla, coconut oil, and pumpkin puree until well combined.

4. Pour batter into the silicone muffin molds and place into the air fryer basket in batches.

5. Cook muffins for 20 minutes.

Nutrition: Calories: 278 protein: 5 g. Fat: 10 g. Carbs: 17 g.

Cappuccino Muffins

Preparation Time:10 minutes

Cooking Time: 20 minutes

Servings:12

Ingredients:

- 4 eggs
- 2 cups almond flour
- 1/2 tsp vanilla
- 1tsp espresso powder
- 1/2 cup sour cream
- 1tsp cinnamon
- 2tsp baking powder
- 1/4 cup coconut flour
- 1/2 cup swerve
- 1/4 tsp salt

Directions:

1. Preheat the air fryer to 325 f.
2. Add sour cream, vanilla, espresso powder, and eggs in a blender and blend until smooth.
3. Add almond flour, cinnamon, baking powder, coconut flour, sweetener, and salt. Blend again until smooth.

4. Pour batter into the silicone muffin molds and place into the air fryer basket. (cook in batches)

5. Cook muffins for 20 minutes.

Nutrition: Calories: 367 Protein: 2 g. Fat: 7 g. Carbs: 10 g.

Moist Cinnamon Muffins

Preparation Time:10 minutes

Cooking Time: 12 minutes

Servings:20

Ingredients:

- 1tbsp cinnamon
- 1tsp baking powder
- 2scoops vanilla protein powder
- 1/2cup almond flour
- 1/2 cup coconut oil
- 1/2 cup pumpkin puree
- 1/2 cup almond butter

Directions:

1. Preheat the air fryer to 325 f.
2. In a large bowl, combine together all dry ingredients and mix well.
3. Add wet Ingredients into the dry ingredients and mix until well combined.
4. Pour batter into the silicone muffin molds and place into the air fryer basket. (cook in batches)
5. Cook muffins for 12 minutes.

Nutrition: Calories: 212 Protein: 7 g. Fat: 8 g. Carbs:

13 g.

Cream Cheese Muffins

Preparation Time:10 minutes

Cooking Time: 16 minutes

Servings:10

Ingredients:

- 2 eggs
- 1/2 cup erythritol
- 8 oz cream cheese
- 1tsp ground cinnamon
- 1/2 tsp vanilla

Directions:

1. Preheat the air fryer to 325 f.
2. In a bowl, mix together cream cheese, vanilla, erythritol, and eggs until soft.
3. Pour batter into the silicone muffin molds and sprinkle cinnamon on top.
4. Place muffin molds into the air fryer basket and cook for 16 minutes.

Nutrition: Calories: 140 Protein: 2 g. Fat: 0 g. Carbs: 5 g.

Strawberry Muffins

Preparation Time:10 minutes

Cooking Time: 15 minutes

Servings:12

Ingredients:

- 3eggs
- 1tsp ground cinnamon
- 2tsp baking powder
- 2 1/2 cups almond flour
- 2/3 cup fresh strawberries, diced
- 1/3 cup heavy cream
- 1tsp vanilla
- 1/2 cup swerve
- 5tbsp butter

Directions:

1. Preheat the air fryer 325 f.
2. Add butter and sweetener in a bowl and beat using a hand mixer until smooth.
3. Add eggs, cream, and vanilla and beat until frothy.
4. In another bowl, sift together almond flour, cinnamon, baking powder, and salt.

5. Add almond flour mixture to wet ingredients and mix until well combined.
6. Add strawberries and fold well.
7. Pour batter into the silicone muffin molds and place into the air fryer basket in batches.
8. Cook muffins for 15 minutes.

Nutrition: Calories: 367 Protein: 2 g. Fat: 7 g. Carbs: 10 g.

Pecan Muffins

Preparation Time:10 minutes

Cooking Time: 15 minutes

Servings:12

Ingredients:

1. 4eggs
2. 1tsp vanilla
3. 1/4cup almond milk
4. 2tbsp butter, melted
5. 1/2 cup swerve
6. 1tsp psyllium husk
7. 1tbsp baking powder
8. 1/2cup pecans, chopped
9. 1/2tsp ground cinnamon
10. 2tsp allspice
11. 11/2 cups almond flour

Instructions:

1. Preheat the air fryer to 370 f.
2. Beat eggs, almond milk, vanilla, sweetener, and butter in a bowl using a hand mixer until smooth.
3. Add remaining ingredients and mix until well combined.

4. Pour batter into the silicone muffin molds and place into the air fryer basket in batches.

5. Cook muffins for 15 minutes.

Nutrition: Calories: 357 Protein: 3 g. Fat: 8 g. Carbs: 12 g.

Blackberry Muffins

Preparation Time:5 minutes

Cooking Time: 12 minutes |

Serves 8

Ingredients:

- ½ cup fresh blackberries
- 1½ cups almond flour
- teaspoon baking powder
- ½ teaspoon baking soda
- ½ cup swerve
- ¼ teaspoon kosher salt
- eggs
- ¼ cup coconut oil, melted
- ½ cup milk
- ½ teaspoon vanilla paste

Directions:

1. Line an 8-cup muffin tin with paper liners.
2. Thoroughly combine the almond flour, salt, swerve, baking powder, and baking soda in a mixing bowl.
3. Whisk together the eggs, milk, vanilla, and coconut oil in a separate mixing bowl until smooth.

4. Add the wet mixture to the dry and fold in the blackberries. Stir with a spatula just until well incorporated.

5. Spoon the batter into the muffin cups, filling each about three- quarters full.

6. Place the muffin tin on the bake position.

7. Select bake, set temperature to 350ºf (180ºc), and set Time to 12 minutes.

8. When done, the tops should be golden and a toothpick inserted in the middle should come out clean.

9. Allow the muffins to cool in the muffin tin for 10 minutes before removing and serving

Nutrition: Calories: 267 Protein: 4 g. Fat: 7 g. Carbs: 8 g.

Lemony Raspberry Muffins

Preparation Time:5 minutes

Cooking Time: 15 minutes

Serves 6

Ingredients:

- 2 cups almond flour
- 3/4cup Swerve
- 1/4teaspoons baking powder
- 1/3teaspoon ground allspice
- 1/3teaspoon ground anise star
- 1/2teaspoon grated lemon zest
- 1/4teaspoon salt
- eggs
- 1 cup sour cream
- 1/2cup coconut oil
- 1/2cup raspberries

Directions:

1. Line a muffin pan with 6 paper liners.
2. In a mixing bowl, mix the almond flour, baking powder, Swerve, lemon zest, allspice, anise, and salt.

3. In another mixing bowl, beat the eggs, coconut oil, and sour cream until well mixed. Add the egg mixture to the flour mixture and stir to combine. Mix in the raspberries.

4. Scrape the batter into the muffin cups, filling each about three-quarters full.

5. Place the muffin pan on the bake position.

6. Select Bake, set temperature to 345ºF (174ºC), and set Time to 15 minutes.

7. When cooking is complete, the tops should be golden and a toothpick inserted in the middle should come out clean.

8. Allow the muffins to cool for 10 minutes in the muffin pan before removing and serving.

Nutrition: Calories: 365 Protein: 2 g. Fat: 9 g. Carbs: 10 g.

Cinnamon Pecan Muffins

Preparation Time:10 minutes

Cooking Time: 15 minutes

Servings:12

Ingredients:

- 4 eggs
- tbsp baking powder
- 1/2 cups almond flour
- 1 tsp vanilla
- 1/4 cup unsweetened almond milk
- 1/2 cup pecans, chopped
- 1/2 tsp ground cinnamon
- tsp allspice
- tbsp butter, melted
- 1/2 cup Swerve
- 1 tsp psyllium husk

Directions:

1. Preheat the cosori air fryer to 400 F.
2. Beat eggs, almond milk, vanilla, sweetener, and butter in a mixing bowl using a hand mixer until smooth.
3. Add remaining ingredients and mix until well combined.

4. Pour batter into silicone muffin molds and
place in the air fryer basket. In batches.
5. Cook for 15 minutes.

Nutrition: Calories 101 Fat 8.9 g Carbohydrates 3.6
g Sugar 0.5 g Protein 3.2 g Cholesterol 60 mg

Strawberry Almond Muffins

Preparation Time:10 minutes

Cooking Time: 20 minutes

Servings:12

Ingredients:

- 3 eggs
- 2 1/2 cups almond flour
- 1/2 cup Swerve
- 5 tbsp butter, melted
- tsp cinnamon
- tsp baking powder
- 2/3 cup strawberries, diced
- 1/3 cup heavy cream
- 1 tsp vanilla
- 1/4 tsp Himalayan salt

Directions:

1. Preheat the cosori air fryer to 350 F.
2. In a bowl, beat together butter and swerve. Add eggs, cream, and vanilla and beat until frothy.
3. Sift together almond flour, cinnamon, baking powder, and salt.

4. Add almond flour mixture to the wet ingredients and mix until combined. Add strawberries and fold well.

5. Pour batter into the silicone muffin molds and place in the air fryer basket. In batches.

6. Cook for 20 minutes.

Nutrition: Calories 108 Fat 10.1 g Carbohydrates 2.7 g Sugar 0.7 g Protein 2.8 g Cholesterol 58 mg

Cinnamon Cream Cheese Muffins

Preparation Time:10 minutes

Cooking Time: 20 minutes

Servings:10

Ingredients:

- 2 eggs
- 1/2 tsp vanilla extract
- 1/2 cup Swerve
- 8 oz cream cheese
- tsp ground cinnamon

Directions:

1. Preheat the cosori air fryer to 350 F.
2. In a bowl, mix together cream cheese, vanilla, Swerve, and eggs until soft.
3. Pour batter into the silicone muffin mold and sprinkle cinnamon on the tops.
4. Place muffin mold in the air fryer basket. In batches.
5. Cook for 20 minutes.

Nutrition: Calories 93 Fat 8.8 g Carbohydrates 1 g Sugar 0.2 g Protein 2.8 g Cholesterol 58 mg

Moist Almond Muffins

Preparation Time:10 minutes

Cooking Time: 15 minutes

Servings:20

Ingredients:

- 1/2 cup coconut oil
- 1/2 cup almond flour
- 1/2 cup pumpkin puree
- 1/2 cup almond butter
- tbsp cinnamon
- tsp baking powder
- scoops vanilla protein powder

Directions:

1. Preheat the cosori air fryer to 350 F.
2. In a large bowl, mix together all dry ingredients.
3. Add wet Ingredients into the dry ingredients and mix until well combined.
4. Pour batter into the silicone muffin molds and place in the air fryer basket. In batches.
5. Cook for 15 minutes.

Nutrition: Calories 68 Fat 6.1 g Carbohydrates 1.2 g

Sugar 0.3 g Protein 3 g Cholesterol 0 mg

Lemon Cheese Muffins

Preparation Time:10 minutes

Cooking Time: 14 minutes

Servings:12

Ingredients:

- 3 eggs
- 1/4 cup coconut oil
- 1/4 cup ricotta cheese
- cup almond flour
- tsp lemon extract
- 1/4 cup heavy cream
- 4 true lemon packets
- tbsp poppy seeds
- 1 tsp baking powder
- 1/3 cup Swerve

Directions:

1. Add all Ingredients into the large mixing bowl and beat until fluffy.
2. Pour batter into the silicone muffin molds and place in the air fryer basket. In batches.
3. Cook at 320 F for 14 minutes or until cooked.

Nutrition: Calories 93 Fat 8.8 g Carbohydrates 1.6 g
Sugar 0.4 g Protein 2.8 g Cholesterol 46 mg

Yummy Brownie Muffins

Preparation Time:10 minutes

Cooking Time: 15 minutes

Servings:6

Ingredients:

- 3 eggs
- 1/3 cup unsweetened cocoa powder
- 1/2 cup Swerve
- cup almond flour
- 1 tbsp gelatin
- 1/3 cup butter, melted

Directions:

1. Add all Ingredients into the mixing bowl and stir until well combined.
2. Pour mixture into the mini silicone muffin molds.
3. Place molds into the air fryer basket and cook at 350 F for 10-15 minutes.

Nutrition: Calories 164 Fat 15.4 g Carbohydrates 4 g Sugar 0.4 g Protein 5.8 g Cholesterol 109 mg

Cheesecake Muffins

Preparation Time:10 minutes

Cooking Time: 20 minutes

Servings:12

Ingredients:

- 2 eggs
- 16 oz cream cheese
- 1/2 tsp vanilla
- 1/2 cup Swerve
- 6 tbsp unsweetened cocoa powder

Directions:

1. Preheat the cosori air fryer to 350 F.
2. In a mixing bowl, beat cream cheese until smooth.
3. Add remaining ingredients and beat until well combined.
4. Spoon mixture into the silicone muffin molds.
5. Place molds in the air fryer basket and cook for 18-20 minutes. Cook in batches.

Nutrition: Calories 149 Fat 14.3 g Carbohydrates 2.6 g Sugar 0.2 g Protein 4.3 g Cholesterol 69 mg

Healthy Blueberry Muffins

Preparation Time:10 Minutes

Cooking Time: 10 Minutes

Servings: 8 to 10

Ingredients:

- 2 teaspoons vanilla extract
- cup blueberries
- ½ teaspoon salt
- cup yogurt
- 1 ½ cups cake flour
- ½ cup sugar
- teaspoons baking powder
- 1/3 cup vegetable oil
- 1 egg

Directions:

1. Place your air fryer on a flat kitchen surface; plug it and turn it on. Set temperature to 355 degrees F and let it preheat for 4-5 minutes.

2. Take 10 muffin molds and gently coat them using a cooking oil or spray.

3. In a bowl of medium size, thoroughly mix the flour, sugar, baking powder and salt.

4. In a bowl of medium size, thoroughly mix the yogurt, oil, egg and vanilla extract. Mix both bowl mixtures. Add the chocolate chips.

5. Add the mixture into muffin molds evenly.

6. Add the molds in the basket. Push the air-frying basket in the air fryer. Cook for 10 minutes.

7. Slide out the basket; serve warm!

Nutrition: Calories - 214 Fat – 8g Carbohydrates – 32g Fiber – 1g Protein – 4g

Kale Egg Muffins

Preparation Time:10 minutes

Cooking Time: 15 minutes

Servings:4

Ingredients:

- 3 eggs
- 1/2 cup kale, chopped
- tsp olive oil
- 1 tbsp onion, minced
- 1/4 cup Swiss cheese, shredded
- 1/2 cup mushrooms, diced
- Pepper
- Salt

Directions:

1. Heat oil in a medium pan over medium-high heat. Add mushrooms and sauté for 2-3 minutes.
2. Add onion and kale and sauté for 2 minutes. Remove pan from heat and set aside to cool.
3. In a bowl, whisk eggs with pepper and salt.
4. Add sautéed mushroom kale mixture and shredded cheese and stir well.

5. Pour egg mixture into the silicone muffin molds.

6. Place molds into the air fryer basket and cook at 350 F for 15 minutes.

7. Serve and enjoy.

Nutrition: Calories 90 Fat 6.4 g Carbohydrates 2 g Sugar 0.6 g Protein 6.5 g Cholesterol 129 mg

Tomato Basil Egg Muffins

Preparation Time:10 minutes

Cooking Time: 20 minutes

Servings:6

Ingredients:

- 6 eggs
- 1/2 tbsp basil, chopped
- tsp olive oil
- 1/2 cup feta cheese, crumbled
- 5 cherry tomatoes, chopped
- sun-dried tomatoes, chopped
- Pepper
- Salt

Directions:

1. In a mixing bowl, whisk eggs with pepper and salt. Add remaining ingredients and stir well.
2. Pour egg mixture into the silicone muffin molds.
3. Place molds into the air fryer basket and cook at 400 F for 20 minutes.
4. Serve and enjoy.

Nutrition: Calories 143 Fat 9 g Carbohydrates 8.1 g

Sugar 5.7 g Protein 9 g Cholesterol 175 mg

Spinach Garlic Egg Muffins

Preparation Time:10 minutes

Cooking Time: 15 minutes

Servings:6

Ingredients:

- 5 eggs
- 1/4 tsp garlic powder
- 1/4 tsp onion powder
- bacon slice, cooked and crumbled
- 1/2 cup mushrooms, chopped
- 1 cup spinach, chopped
- Pepper
- Salt

Directions:

1. In a mixing bowl, whisk eggs with garlic powder, onion powder, pepper, and salt. Stir in spinach, mushrooms, and bacon.
2. Pour egg mixture into the six silicone muffin molds.
3. Place molds into the air fryer basket and cook at 400 F for 15 minutes.
4. Serve and enjoy.

Nutrition: Calories 73 Fat 5 g Carbohydrates 0.9 g

Sugar 0.5 g Protein 6.1 g Cholesterol 140 mg